THE NEXT PROJECT

The Economics of U.S. Healthcare and A Better Way Forward for the American People

STU RODNICK

This book is dedicated to:

My mom and dad, for teaching me the importance of decency.

Table of Contents

Introduction

We are only 20 years into this century, and we've witnessed the shattering of the dot-com economy, 9/11, the financial crisis of 2007, and the COVID-19 pandemic. It's tough to keep up with all this change, and trying to starts to feel like looking out of a car window during a hailstorm. It is impossible to know what lies around the corner.

This project is a collection of essays about the economics of U.S. Healthcare, with an emphasis on making it better for the masses. It focuses on the long-term trends that have been in place prior to COVID-19, trends that will continue to be in place after COVID-19 unless we utilize the current crisis as a wake-up call to make lasting changes to the healthcare system. COVID-19 has made the inequities at the core of the healthcare system more transparent, and at the heart of these essays is the belief that there are enough good-souled, compassionate people out there who want the healthcare system to be better for all. We need to make that happen.

Quoting President Franklin Roosevelt, "In our seeking for economic and political progress as a nation, we all go up, or else we all go down, as one people." This statement is ever applicable to the United States of today, especially as it relates to securing access to affordable healthcare for everybody.

A couple of facts. The United States is the wealthiest country in the world. The United States has the largest population of any rich nation in the world. The United States spends way more on healthcare per person than any other nation. Yet, the United States found a way to have a greater percentage of uninsured people than just about every other developed economy.

The most incredible parts of U.S. healthcare are the great people who provide the *care* in healthcare, the bioscientists who led so many drug discoveries, and the ingenuity of all the medical device technology that didn't exist 20 years ago. Yet the U.S. healthcare system that is full of so much greatness is at the same time full of the challenges of a system caught between public health needs and unchecked, non-transparent pricing.

The World's Greatest Advancement: Longevity

The greatest achievement from the last 100 years or so is longevity, the massive extension of the human lifespan. From 1900 to 2000, lifespans in the United States increased 62%.

If you were born in the United States in 1900, you were expected to live to 47; if you were born in the United States in 2000, your life expectation rose to 77. As the medical profession shifted from opinion-based approaches to the science and data-based treatments of the 20th century, 30 additional years of life were discovered.

Compared to how much time was afforded to people born in 1900, this equates to a lot more time to take in the world. That said, with that extra time we also found a bunch of modern problems people didn't contend with when they only lived to 47.

So, thanks to longevity for offering up all the time to work with, even if we are still in a rush all too often. This rush could include honking the horn within two seconds of a traffic light turning green or growing impatient when our high-speed internet seems slow, or when we are down to one or two bars of mobile receptivity. We've all been there.

When people lived to 47, they didn't worry about that kind of stuff.

Talkin' About an Aging Revolution

As the senior population in the United States grows into a massive-sized population, we are experiencing an aging revolution. This places us in uncharted territory. We have little idea how such a large number of people will fill all their time, or how they will care for themselves.

Some people's retirements will last as long or even longer than their careers, something that slipped by the pension actuaries last century. Longevity wasn't in their models.

Actuaries didn't expect people to live such long lives today. People beat the modelers.

The probabilities of life now say that a 65-year-old female has a 34% chance of living to 90 while a 65-year-old male has a 22% chance of living to 90. In present day America, a 65-year-old female can expect to live to 85 and a 65-year-old male can expect to live to 83.

It wasn't that long ago that life expectancy in the United States was still hovering around 65. Babies born in 1942 represented the first babies to arrive in the world with a life expectancy greater than 65. Back then, living to 65 was considered a full life. So much has since changed.

To put the size of the senior population in perspective, let's work with some history and numbers. In just a few years, there will be more seniors in the United States than there will be people of any age in the entire United Kingdom.

It is expected that there will be more than 73 million Americans over the age of 65 in 2030. By then, the entire population of the United Kingdom will be around 70 million. Quite a change for a country that was once just a small colonial territory that belonged to the folks across the pond. In 1776, the 13 colonies had a total population of around 2.5 million people, while the United Kingdom had a population of around 8 million people.

Thanks to the aging revolution, a 65-year-old today can be considered, in many ways, as young as a 45-year-old in the 1940s. Each could look forward to having around 20 more years to take in the goodness of the world. This makes 65 still young in today's world.

Hacking the Data of a Longer Life

Paying attention to how the leading causes of death have changed over the years offers some of the best healthcare guidance, guidance that hopefully increases the odds of living a longer life.

In 1900, the three leading causes of death in the United States were pneumonia and the flu (they were grouped together in 1900), tuberculosis, and gastro infections. This was before the world had access to penicillin and other antibiotics and vaccinations.

Heart disease, which had been the leading cause of death just about every year since 1910, was just the fourth leading cause of death in 1900. This isn't surprising. It was rare for people to live beyond 50 back then, and heart disease tends to manifest later on in life. That said, the only time heart disease hasn't been the leading cause of death since 1910 was from 1918–1920, the years of the 1918 Flu Pandemic.

As lifespans increased throughout the century, the leading causes of death changed with the times. In

2000, the three leading causes of death from illnesses in the United States were heart disease, cancer, and strokes. The leading causes of death among the senior population were the same as the overall population.

By 2018, the top two causes of death in the United States remained heart disease and cancer, accounting for 44% of all deaths in the country. They have consistently ranked as the top two causes of death since the 1940s. Lower respiratory diseases (including asthma) were the third leading cause of death. Similar to 2000, the leading causes of death among the senior population remained the same as the general population in 2018.

By the time the data is available from 2020, COVID-19 will be among the top three causes of death in 2020. A notable change, considering that the last time the leading causes of death changed this suddenly was during the 1918 Flu Pandemic.

The Fifth Largest Economy in the World, U.S. Healthcare

The United States economy led the world in 2018, with the value of all the goods and services produced (GDP) in the U.S. reaching a value of $20.5 trillion. This represents 24% of the global economy. A staggering sum, recognizing only around 4% of the world's population resides in the U.S.

Total healthcare expenditures in the United States were $3.6 trillion in 2018. This results in healthcare expenditures representing 18% of the U.S. economy and 4% of the $86 trillion global economy. Of the $3.6 trillion spent on healthcare in the United States, government payments were responsible for approximately 45% of the total.

It will be nearly two years before we will know the full extent of how economic activity and healthcare costs were impacted by COVID-19. However, it's certain that 2020 will stand out as a unique historical time, which means the years before COVID-19 will offer a more transparent portrayal of how healthcare costs have trended during recent times.

The amount of money spent on healthcare in the United States has grown so enormous that if the U.S. healthcare industry were its own national economy, it would rank as the fifth largest economy in the world, trailing only the economies of the United States, China, Germany, and Japan.

It is hard to grapple with the fact that $1 out of every $5 spent in the United States is for a healthcare-related expense, while $1 out of every $25 spent throughout the world is for a healthcare-related expense in the United States.

The Accidental System of Care in the U.S.

As of 2018, about half (55%) of America's population has health insurance connected to their employer or the employer of a family member. This figure was closer to two-thirds (64%) of Americans in 2000, and as of this year the numbers are trending closer to two out of every five (45%) Americans having employer-sponsored health insurance due to the impact of COVID-19 on the economy and labor market. Besides employer-sponsored health insurance, the largest sources of healthcare coverage in the United States are Medicare and Medicaid.

As common as employer-sponsored health insurance is, few people are familiar with the origins of private health insurance. Given the economic uncertainty of COVID-19, that people are living longer, and that people have way more career turns than prior generations, it is now much more important to understand how private insurance came about.

Employer-sponsored health insurance plans were introduced during World War II, when many Americans were serving overseas. This led to a workforce shortage back home. In response, companies bid up salaries, leading to a chaotic situation in which many other companies couldn't afford to staff up. In response, Franklin Roosevelt signed the Economic Stabilization Act of 1942, which forbade businesses from raising pay during the war.

With the wage freeze in place and war raging, businesses focused on other benefits with which they could entice employees. Employer-sponsored health insurance was one of these new benefits, helping employer-sponsored plans gain quick adoption.

Then, shortly after the employer-sponsored plan's introductions, health insurance costs became a full tax deduction for businesses. This provided further incentive for companies to offer health insurance to their workers.

Over time, the adoption of the employer-sponsored health insurance plans ushered in the growth of the insurance market. In 1940, just 9% of Americans had health insurance, while by 1960 more than two-thirds of Americans had health insurance.

While employer-sponsored healthcare was a brilliant idea during World War II, now, eight decades after World War II started, the needs of Americans have changed, and it has become an outdated approach. Largely, this is because people used to have lifetime employment with their employers, whereas people of today switch jobs much more often. People born between 1957 and 1964 held an average of 12 jobs between when they were 18 and 52, a number that will surely increase over the coming years. More job changes results in people also having to change their insurance coverage far more often than prior generations.

It also means insurance companies have less incentive to focus on people's long-term health, since by the time people grow old, their coverage will be provided by another insurance carrier or the government.

If private insurance companies' shortsighted view of long-term health isn't enough reason to deemphasize the role of employer-sponsored health insurance plans, consider it from another perspective: employers.

Employers really don't want to fund healthcare insurance for their workers because it has grown into one of the biggest costs of operating a business. In the words of Warren Buffett, "The ballooning costs of health care act as a hungry tapeworm on the American economy."

2020 will represent the first time in seven decades that less than half of America's population has health coverage through employers, and the first time ever that government payments will represent more than 50% of the healthcare expenditures in the United States.

This makes now the ideal time to reform the healthcare system so it fits better into a world that has changed so much since World War II.

If Wages Rose Like Health Insurance Premiums

The annual premium for an employer-sponsored health insurance plan for American families was $20,576 in 2019, increasing from $5,791 in 1999. Since employers fund around 70% of the health insurance premiums, the portion of the premiums that workers were responsible for was $6,172 in 2019. For perspective, recognize that $6,172 is more than the entire plan's cost just 20 years ago.

In a backdrop where the real (inflation adjusted) median household income increased 3% from 2000–2018, it's not a favorable equation for American households that their insurance costs increased 255%. It significantly reduces their take-home pay, as a much greater share of income is absorbed by insurance premiums.

The steep rise in health insurance premiums magnifies how much influence the health insurance industry has gained. The largest health insurance companies—United Healthcare, Aetna, Anthem, Cigna, and Humana—collectively generated around $516 billion in revenue during 2019, representing a lot of money to spend on behalf of policy holders.

Since the insurance industry ultimately decides which services and medicines patients are covered for, along with what costs patients are responsible for, the industry has developed a powerful role in determining how American healthcare evolves. This leaves the insurance industry to make bigger and bigger decisions about the direction that U.S. healthcare takes.

Very surprisingly, the increased purchasing clout of large health insurance companies hasn't held back healthcare costs. Per capita healthcare costs paid through private insurance increased 53% between 2008 and 2018, compared to an increase of just 22% for healthcare costs paid through Medicare.

This demonstrates how much health insurance has contributed to the exorbitant healthcare pricing environment that has become a cornerstone of healthcare in the United States.

The Complex World of University Healthcare Systems

Hospitals represented around a third of the healthcare costs in the United States in 2018, making hospitals by far the largest part of the United States healthcare system.

Between 2000 and 2018, hospital expenditures in the United States increased 287%, from $415 billion in 2000 to $1.2 trillion in 2018. This is unquestionably a lot of money. To put it in perspective, the total healthcare expenditures in the United States were just $1.4 trillion in 2000, slightly more than was spent at just hospitals during 2018.

One of the biggest changes in the hospital landscape during recent times is that small teaching hospitals and community hospitals have increasingly become part of mega-sized university healthcare systems. University healthcare systems have grown so massive that, as an example, when watching baseball games it's increasingly common for the advertisements behind home plate to feature a university-affiliated hospital system. These are the same advertisements that have traditionally featured mass-market brands like Budweiser or McDonald's.

University-affiliated healthcare systems have grown so huge that university healthcare systems have increasingly become the largest sources of revenue for schools and even entire state school systems.

For example, across the University of California system, health services revenues (which includes all of the hospital systems, clinics, and doctors affiliated with the state's different campuses) increased from 27% of the university system's revenues in 2010 to 33% in 2019. Health services revenues grew from $5.9 billion in 2010 to $12.8 billion in 2019. A similar story exists at many other universities across the country. The portion of revenue generated from medical services was 44% at the University of Texas, 58% at Stanford, 24% at the University of Colorado, and 24% at Yale during the year of their most recent financial reports.

Based on the current trajectory, many universities will become more akin to holding companies that include a healthcare system and a teaching university, a big difference from the past when teaching universities were affiliated with relatively small, local hospitals.

As the revenue from universities' medical systems eclipse the revenue from the more traditional academic parts of the universities, such as tuition, it demonstrates how complicated the economics of healthcare have become.

Of course, it is even more complicated now that the universities are running healthcare systems during the pandemic, while the rest of their campuses are closed.

The Piñata of Healthcare: The Pharmaceutical Industry

The pharmaceutical industry has grown into the piñata of rising healthcare costs, since in the complex world of healthcare, prescription drugs are actually one of the more transparent costs. With more than 4 billion retail prescriptions filled each year, people have lots of opportunities to think about the costs of prescription medicines.

Overall, the retail pharmaceutical industry represents approximately 9% of healthcare expenditures in the U.S. When you include specialty drugs, which are administered in hospitals and doctors' offices, pharmaceutical's share of health expenditures in the United States rises to 17%.

In comparison, hospital costs comprise 33% of healthcare expenditures. However, while just about everybody takes at least one medicine during a given year, only around 7% of Americans require an overnight stay in a hospital and just one in five people visit an emergency room during a typical year. Of course, 2020 is atypical due to COVID-19.

With so few people requiring the services of a hospital and so many people requiring prescription medicine, the pharmaceutical industry is a much more visible target for runaway medical costs than rarely visited hospitals

A lot of the resentment toward the pharmaceutical industry is deserved. It is an industry that has seen more than its share of abusive companies manipulate the patent system or introduce highly awaited new products with excessively high price points. These high price points limit access among patients most in need of the medicines. The industry also grossly overcharges Americans for products that are far cheaper in other parts of the world. It operates in devious ways and invests boatloads of money in lobbying to prevent the world from changing. It's an industry that has done more than its share of work to earn the disdain of Americans.

Case in point, the jaw-dropping list prices that pharmaceutical companies set for their products, list prices that are as fictitious as the room rates published on the back of hotel doors. Nobody pays the back of the door price for a hotel room, and hopefully the same can be said for the list prices of pharmaceutical products.

This explains why 79% of people believe prescription medicines are priced unreasonably. It is a market that people are hoping changes its ways.

The Pharmaceutical Industry's Conundrum

The United States government is the pharmaceutical industry's best customer. In fact, it is the industry's best customer in the entire world.

Through a combination of Medicare, Medicaid, Veterans Affairs, Department of Defense, and Children's Health Insurance Programs, the U.S. government represents nearly half of the pharmaceutical industry's revenues in the United States, the industry's largest market. That the industry's best customer has had its negotiating leverage limited highlights the impracticality of how drug pricing works.

In most industries, the biggest customer should be commanding the lowest price per unit. However, this isn't how it works with drug pricing. Case in point, Medicare is the largest of the government programs, yet it can't directly negotiate drug prices.

To understand why Medicare can't negotiate better pricing for pharmaceuticals, you need to travel back to 2003. That's when retail pharmaceutical benefits were first included in the Medicare program. This took place through the passing of a bill known as the Medicare Prescription Drug Modernization Program.

As the Prescription Drug Modernization Program bill made its way through congress, the pharmaceutical industry channeled all of its lobbying might (big, big bucks) to prevent the government from gaining the ability to negotiate drug prices for the large and massively growing Medicare population.

This was a costly and unnecessary giveaway to the industry. When the Medicare Prescription Drug Modernization Program was introduced in 2003, there were only around 36 million seniors in the United States; today, there are approximately 56 million seniors. Also, it is important to point out that Medicare also provides coverage for around 9 million disabled Americans who qualify for Medicare.

It was easy to see in 2003 that Medicare's drug tally was going to become an enormous cost. Seniors fill more than twice as many prescriptions as the rest of the population, and so of course, as the senior population ages and grows in size, far more prescriptions need to be filled.

In 2006, a few years after the act was passed, Medicare's share of retail drug spending was 18%. By 2018, this would increase to 32%. Between the many cost increases for pharmaceutical products and a larger Medicare population, Americans have been overcharged in excess of a trillion dollars for pharmaceutical products compared to the prices paid in other rich countries.

The widespread recognition of medicine's high costs results in 92% of democrats, 90% of independents, and 85% of republicans favoring granting the government the ability to negotiate drug prices for the Medicare population.

Many in the pharmaceutical industry counter this proposition with the argument that the high drug prices are necessary to support innovation. It's an outdated argument. The reality is that there isn't a better, more utopian market to innovate for than a soon-to-be 73 million seniors in the wealthiest country in the world, which is what the size of the senior population is expected to be in 2030.

Accessing Medicine Like the Rest of the World

While the United States spends more on prescription drugs than every other country in the world, the U.S. doesn't spend that much more, as a percentage of the overall economy, on prescription drugs as some other rich countries do.

Prescription drugs represent around 2% of the United States economy, compared to 1.7% of Switzerland's, 2% of Japan's, and 1.8% of Canada's economies. The big difference between the U.S. and these other nations is that America spends more on individual prescriptions than other countries do. The other rich nations achieve greater purchasing power and better pricing than the United States.

As an example, look at the price of insulin. It averages $34.75 a dose in the United States while costing an average of $10.58 across a basket of 11 developed economies. Or look at Humira, the top-selling drug in the world: it costs $2,346 a dose in the U.S. compared to an average of $451 across the same basket of 11 developed economies. In an age of global supply chains, pharmaceutical products are increasingly manufactured outside the United States, while the prices paid for medicines greatly varies throughout the world.

It's illogical that the pharmaceutical industry can manufacture products outside the U.S. and import finished products, yet it's illegal for patients to purchase drugs from international markets, where the products are cheaper. Either way, the products have to be inspected before they enter the United States.

If the prices paid for medicines in the United States was similar to the prices paid in other developed economies, and the share of GDP that the U.S. spends on pharmaceuticals held steady at around 2%, it would be a big win for the U.S. healthcare system.

This would result in lower drug prices and achieve the very important outcome of expanding access to medicine. With lower drug prices, adherence rates will be higher, which prevents the need for far more costly hospital visits.

By offering lower price points and expanding access to medicines, both patients and the drug industry would win. To understand why, look to an example from outside the field of medicine. When the Atlanta

Falcons built a new stadium, the team reduced the price of popular food and beverages choices by 50%. The result is the team saw concession sales spike 16%. This is an example far from the world of medicine, but business is business and the pharmaceutical industry would reap similar sales gains by increasing access to medicines.

Simply put, shifting to a price times volume business approach would result in greater revenue for the drug companies and would represent a much better solution for all those in need of medicines.

Ode to the Bioscientists
Fighting Cancer

So much progress has been made in reducing the number of deaths from heart disease that the leading causes of death are on the cusp of experiencing a lasting change.

With all the progress in combating heart disease, in 2016 it fell to the second leading cause of death in 23 states, where cancer has become the leading cause of death. Back in 2000, there were only two states where more people died from cancer than heart disease.

Before the COVID-19 outbreak, cancer was projected to surpass heart disease as the leading cause of death in the United States by 2020. For context, in 2018, the latest year data is available, 655,381 people passed away from heart disease while 599,294 people passed away from cancer.

As cancer turns into the leading cause of death in the country, we are very fortunate that more medical progress is being made to combat cancer than ever before. Many of the brightest minds in the world are currently developing treatments and cures for different types of cancer.

The field of immuno-oncology, which focuses on developing new approaches and medicines to attack cancer, is experiencing magical progress. As of 2017, over 2,004 immuno-oncology drugs targeting a total of 303 different variations of cancer were in testing.

All the activity in the field of immuno-oncology highlights the promise that drug treatments can offer. This is so important during any period of time, however these advancements feel even more special right now, as the world is facing such a challenging global health crisis. It makes medical progress even more important.

A quote I heard a while back speaks to a world full of medical advancement and hope. Larry Fink, honcho of the ginormous asset management firm BlackRock, said in an interview, "What was once a terminal illness is now a chronic condition."

This quote captures the magic of medicine in the modern world. What used to be considered a terminal health condition can now increasingly be managed with the help of modern medicine. Hats off to the bioscientists of the world.

The $2 Trillion Healthcare Bill

B y 2030, the cost to provide healthcare to seniors will reach $2 trillion per year. It's simple and conservative math. There will be 73 million seniors, and their average healthcare costs will be approximately $30,000 per person annually.

This may not seem like a conservative estimate, but let's look at the math. As of 2010, the average annual healthcare costs for seniors was $18,424. If these costs increased just 2.5% each year from 2010 to 2030, then seniors' average annual healthcare costs will reach $30,000 per year in 2030.

All this adds up to total healthcare costs for the senior population surpassing $2.1 trillion by 2030. This makes it clear that we are going to require better thought-out public health policies to match the needs of a massive aging population.

Coming up with solutions isn't going to be easy, though, especially since when it comes to healthcare, ten years down the road is as good as right around the corner. It takes time to gain support for new policies and implement changes.

So while none of this should be a surprise to anybody by the time 2030 rolls in, there is an incredibly strong likelihood that it will surprise nearly everybody. Ten years isn't a luxurious amount of time to produce meaningful solutions when it involves the healthcare system.

Hopefully, the crossroad of COVID-19 can result in new policies and reforms to be rolled out quicker than they would be in more ordinary times. The dollars here are so large that if we can find ways to spend 25% less per person without compromising access to care, it will save $500 billion per year. Too big of an opportunity to chuck on down the road.

The Big Bucks Separating U.S. Healthcare from the Rest of the World

Healthcare is much more expensive in the U.S. than anywhere else in the world. While the per capita healthcare spending among countries that are a part of the Organization for Economic Co-operation & Development (OECD), a consortium of 37 developed (rich) economies, was $3,994 in 2018, it was $11,172 per person in the United States. In other words, healthcare costs nearly three times more in the U.S. than it does in the rest of the world.

But OK, if healthcare was three times more expensive per person in the U.S., and lifespans are longer, there would be some logic supporting the high costs. However, the life expectancy in the United States is 78.7, compared to an average of 80.6 across the developed world.

In fact, the United States not only tops the world in per capita healthcare expenditures, there isn't even a close second. Switzerland, which spends $7,316 per person on healthcare, is the country with the second highest healthcare spend per person. There isn't a rational answer for why the U.S. spends 53% more on healthcare per person than a super wealthy nation such as Switzerland.

To get a sense of the healthcare expenses in other countries, the per capita healthcare costs were $4,974 in Canada, $4,766 in Japan, $4,069 in the U.K., and $2,779 in Israel. It is perplexing to grapple with the fact that healthcare costs are so much more expensive in the U.S., because each of these other countries has a longer life expectancy than America. Life expectancies are 83.6 in Switzerland, 82.0 in Canada, 84.2 in Japan, 81.3 in the United Kingdom, and 82.6 in Israel.

It's important to call out the fact that the U.S. is a much larger country than all the other OECD nations (China and India aren't members). The large population does add complexity, since there are a lot more people to care for. For example, the population of a given demographic cohort in the U.S. (i.e. region, ethnicity, age-group) is commonly larger than the entire populations of other countries.

However, given that the U.S. is a much larger country than each of the other OECD member countries, it should have greater economies of scale to spread costs across the population. Unfortunately, the economies of scale never surface, and the U.S. spends 2.8 times more per person on healthcare than the other wealthy nations.

Healthcare Around the World

Healthcare systems throughout the developed world share one trait. All of the healthcare systems, with the exception of the United States healthcare system, feature universal health coverage, meaning countries' entire populations have access to healthcare. As of 2018, however, 9.4% of Americans lacked healthcare coverage. Let's take a quick tour of international healthcare systems.

In the United Kingdom, healthcare costs represent 10% of the economy. The government-funded system, the National Health Service (NHS), provides healthcare for the entire population. This results in minimal out-of-pocket costs for the British people. The NHS came about after World War II, when the British deemed it important to provide healthcare for the entire population. The NHS has since become a symbol of national pride in the U.K.

Onward to Switzerland, home of the second-best life expectancy in the world. In Switzerland, healthcare costs represent 12% of the economy. The Swiss system legally requires people to maintain health insurance through what is called the Mandatory Health Insurance system. As part of the Mandatory Health Insurance System, coverage is offered through private insurance companies. The insurance companies receive pricing guidance from the government and must operate in a profit-neutral manner. This lowers the risk of insurance companies holding back access to medical services to increase profits.

Over to Israel, where healthcare costs represent 8% of the economy. In 1995, Israel created a national health system. Israel was the second-to-last developed nation to implement universal healthcare for its population (this leaves the United States as the last holdout). Israel's healthcare system provides health services for nearly all citizens (the military has a separate plan). Israel's National Health Insurance system is administered by four non-profit insurance companies. The government decides which treatments are included in the insurance plans and what reimbursement rates are acceptable. Israel also has a national Electronic Health Record that is way ahead of the rest of the world, and it has been an early pioneer in deploying AI to develop healthcare solutions.

To the far east. Japan has the highest life expectancy in the world. In Japan, healthcare represents 11% of the economy. Basic healthcare insurance is legally required in Japan by what is known as the Statutory Health Insurance System. Insurance is offered through 3,400 insurers and it is funded through a combination of employers and the government. The government maintains the important role of setting insurance prices and the costs of healthcare services, which helps to keep costs in check.

Northward to Canada, where healthcare costs represent 11% of the economy. Canada has a single-payer universal healthcare system that is provided and managed within each of the ten provinces. The system, which is known as Medicare, provides basic coverage for all Canadians.

This all points to a lot of examples of what works across the world, and it offers valuable lessons that can help make the U.S. healthcare system better. From the U.K. and Canada, we see how their governments run single-payer healthcare systems and keep a lid on pricing. From the Swiss, we can see how a healthcare system with government-set pricing and private insurance can efficiently operate. From Israel, we can see how their national Electronic Health Record improves care and reduces duplicative procedures.

From Japan, we can see that the government maintains a strong handle on costs by setting insurance rates and the maximum medical costs that patients are responsible for.

Healthcare systems from across the world provide lots of examples of what works, and these real-life examples can help to reduce the high cost of healthcare in the United States. In challenging times, when the world is in flux, there is a greater opening to deploy big new solutions to old, long-running problems.

Conclusion

The most pragmatic path forward for healthcare in America is to strengthen the Medicare program and make it available to all Americans.

The expansion of Medicare across the entire population removes layers of complexity that have become emblematic of the U.S. healthcare system. Medicaid, Children's Health Insurance Program (CHIP), and the Affordable Care Act (ACA) marketplaces could be consolidated into Medicare and private business would no longer need to provide employer-sponsored insurance plans to employees.

Providing Medicare to all Americans doesn't mean insurance would be eliminated. Insurance companies have a sizable role in Medicare through supplemental and advantage plans. And if employers choose, they can continue to offer sponsored group plans and services as a benefit to their employees.

Some argue they wouldn't want the government to have such a large influence in the healthcare market. However, it already does.

By 2030, government is paced to fund 48% of the healthcare expenditures in the country (up from 36% in 2000). Households are projected to fund 27% of healthcare costs by this time and private businesses are projected to fund 18% of healthcare costs.

As the government has become the biggest purchaser of healthcare services and products, the healthcare system is at a crossroads.

The choices are to fix the whole system or continue to introduce one-off improvements, such as the 2003 decision to add prescription drug coverage to Medicare (which proved to be ineffective at controlling costs) or the 2010 ACA marketplaces (which has proven to be complex).

These one-off patches aren't effective at accounting for how quickly the world is changing. This makes overhauling the entire system the better path forward. It offers the opportunity to construct a healthcare system that's a bright example of America's adaptability and ingenuity.

Looking forward, in 2030 there will be 73 million seniors in the U.S., approximately 125 million people under 65 lacking employee-sponsored healthcare coverage, and a labor force that is on pace to fund more and more of their healthcare insurance costs. It will also be a decade filled with AI and machine learning-led automation which will redefine labor.

These trends and changes point to a decreasing share of people with employer-sponsored coverage, a decline that is entering its fifth decade. The percentage of the population under 65 who have health coverage from an employer-sponsored plan declined from a peak of 79% in 1980 to 61% as of 2018.

To get ahead of 2030, bolstering Medicare is of the highest priority. This can be accomplished by placing greater emphasis on preventative primary care, the deployment of technology to support aging at home, and data analytics to reduce duplicative tests and fraudulent billing.

After bolstering Medicare; Medicaid, CHIP and the ACA marketplaces can be consolidated into Medicare. Medicare's

increased participation and scale can then help to secure better negotiated hospital, provider, testing, and pharmaceutical rates.

These are savings that support the expansion of Medicare and also increased access to treatments. Medicare premiums can then be established based upon household income. People will have the assurance that they'll always have healthcare coverage, and employers will be freed from having to be involved in funding healthcare coverage.

As healthcare has become the defining issue of these times, as a nation we can rise to the occasion so the America of the future is about life, liberty, and the pursuit of happiness *and* healthcare.

Bibliography

Introduction

OECD. 2020. "Health Spending: Indicator." Accessed June 1, 2020. https://data.oecd.org/healthres/health-spending.htm

—. 2020. "Social Protection. "Accessed June 1, 2020. https://stats.oecd.org/Index.aspx?DataSetCode=HEALTH_PROT

Roosevelt, Franklin. n.d. "Franklin Roosevelt Presidency, 1937: Second Inaugural." Joint Congressional Committee on Inaugural Ceremonies (website). Accessed on July 8, 2020. https://www.inaugural.senate.gov/about/past-inaugural-ceremonies/38th-inaugural-ceremonies/

United States Census Bureau. n.d. "U.S. and World Population Clock." Accessed June 1, 2020. https://www.census.gov/popclock/world

World's Greatest Advancement: Longevity

Arias, Elizabeth and Xu, Jiaquin. 2019. "United States Life Tables: 2017." PDF file, *National Vital Statistics Reports* 68, no. 7 (June).

Talkin' About an Aging Revolution

Arias, Elizabeth and Xu, Jiaquin. 2019. "United States Life Tables: 2017." *National Vital Statistics Reports* 68, no. 7 (June).

Encyclopedia.com. 2020. "Populations of Great Britain and America." Last modified May 17, 2020. https://www.encyclopedia.com/history/encyclopedias-almanacs-transcripts-and-maps/populations-great-britain-and-america

Hamilton Project. 2015. "Probability of a 65-Year-Old Living to a Given Age, by Sex and Year." Last modified June 23, 2015. https://www.hamiltonproject.org/charts/probability_of_a_65_year_old_living_to_a_given_age_by_sex_and_year

Office for National Statistics. 2019. "National Population Projections: 2018-Based." Last modified October 21, 2019. https://www.ons.gov.uk/peoplepopulationandcommunity/populationandmigration/population

projections/bulletins/nationalpopulationprojecti
ons/2018based

Social Security Administration. n.d. "Actuarial Life
Table: 2017." Accessed June 8, 2020.
https://www.ssa.gov/oact/STATS/table4c6.htm
l

United States Census Bureau. n.d. "Table 2: Projected
Age and Sex Composition of the Population."
Excel file, 2017 National Population
Projections Tables. Accessed June 8, 2020.
https://www.census.gov/data/tables/2017/demo
/popproj/2017-summary-tables.html

Hacking the Data of a Longer Life

Anderson, Robert. 2002. "Death: Leading Causes for
2000." PDF file, *National Vital Statistics
Report* 50, no. 16 (September).

Centers for Disease Control and Prevention. n.d.
"Leading Causes of Death, 1900–1998." PDF
file. Accessed June 1, 2020.
https://www.cdc.gov/nchs/data/dvs/lead1900_9
8.pdf

Centers for Disease Control and Prevention. 2019. "10
Leading Causes of Death by Age Group,
United States – 2018." Last Modified July 10,
2020.

https://www.cdc.gov/injury/wisqars/LeadingCa
uses.html

Xu, Jiaquan, Sherry L. Murphy, Kenneth D.
Kochanek, and Elizabeth Arias. n.d. "NCHS
Data Brief: Mortality in the United States,
2018." PDF file, Centers for Disease Control
and Prevention. Accessed June 8, 2020.
https://www.cdc.gov/nchs/products/databriefs/
db355.htm

The Fifth Largest Economy in The World

Ballmer, Steve. 2020. "A Letter to Our Country's
Shareholders." USAFacts (website). Last
modified April 17, 2020.
https://usafacts.org/annual-
publications/2020/government-10-k/

Bureau of Economic Analysis. 2019. "Gross Domestic
Product, Fourth Quarter and Annual 2018
(Initial Estimate)." Last modified February 28,
2019. https://www.bea.gov/news/2019/initial-
gross-domestic-product-4th-quarter-and-
annual-2018

Centers for Medicare & Medicaid Services. n.d.
"National Health Expenditures: 2018
Highlights." PDF file. Accessed June 8, 2020.
https://www.cms.gov/files/document/highlight
s.pdf

HowMuch.net. 2019. "The World's $86 Trillion Economy Visualized in One Chart." Last modified August 15, 2019. https://howmuch.net/articles/the-world-economy-2018

United States Census Bureau. n.d. "U.S. and World Population Clock." Accessed June 1, 2020. https://www.census.gov/popclock/world

The Accidental System of Care in the U.S.

Berkshire Hathaway. 2018. "Amazon, Berkshire Hathaway and JPMorgan Chase & Co. to partner on U.S. employee healthcare." Berkshire Hathaway Press Release. January 30, 2018. https://www.berkshirehathaway.com/news/jan3018.pdf

Carroll, Aaron E. 2017. "The Real Reason the U.S. Has Employee Sponsored Health Insurance." The New York Times (website). Last modified September 5, 2017. https://www.nytimes.com/2017/09/05/upshot/the-real-reason-the-us-has-employer-sponsored-health-insurance.html

Centers for Medicare & Medicaid Service. 2019. "National Health Expenditure Data: Historical." Last modified December 17, 2019.

https://www.cms.gov/Research-Statistics-Data-and-Systems/Statistics-Trends-and-Reports/NationalHealthExpendData/NationalHealthAccountsHistorical

Lindquist, Rick. 2014. "Part 1: The History of U.S. Employer-Provided Health Insurance – Post-World War I." Peoplekeep (website). Last modified June 5, 2014. https://www.peoplekeep.com/blog/part-1-the-history-of-u.s.-employer-provided-health-insurance-post-world-war-ii

U.S. Bureau of Labor Statistics. 2019. "Number of Jobs, Labor Market Experience, and Earnings Growth: Results from A National Longitudinal Survey." Last modified August 22, 2019. https://www.bls.gov/news.release/nlsoy.nr0.htm

United States Census Bureau. n.d. "Figure 1: Percentage of People by Type of Health Insurance Coverage and Change From 2017 to 2018." PDF file. Accessed June 8, 2020. https://www.census.gov/content/dam/Census/library/visualizations/2019/demo/p60-267/Figure_1.pdf

—. n.d. "Type of Health Insurance and Coverage Status, All People: 1999 and 2000." Accessed June 8, 2020. https://www2.census.gov/programs-surveys/demo/tables/p60/215/hi00t1.txt

If Wages Rose Like Health Insurance Premiums

Cigna. n.d. "Cigna 2019 Annual Report." PDF file. Accessed June 8, 2020. https://www.cigna.com/static/www-cigna-com/docs/about-us/investor-relations/cigna-2019-annual-report.pdf

CVS. n.d. "2019 Annual Report." PDF file. Accessed June 8, 2020. https://s2.q4cdn.com/447711729/files/doc_financials/2019/annual/FINAL-CVS-AR-bookmarked.pdf

Federal Reserve Bank of St. Louis. 2019. "Real Median Household Income in the United States." Last modified September 10, 2019. https://fred.stlouisfed.org/series/MEHOINUSA672N/

Kaiser Family Foundation. 2019. "2019 Employer Health Benefits Survey." Last modified September 25, 2019. https://www.kff.org/report-section/ehbs-2019-section-1-cost-of-health-insurance/

Kamal, Rabah, Daniel McDermott, and Cynthia Cox. 2019. "How Has U.S. Spending on Healthcare Changed Over Time?" Peterson-KFF Health System Tracker. Last modified December 20, 2019.

https://www.healthsystemtracker.org/chart-collection/u-s-spending-healthcare-changed-time/#item-start

Popa, Rachel. 2020. "5 Largest Health Insurance Companies by Membership." Becker's ASC Review (website). Last modified February 13, 2020. https://www.beckersasc.com/asc-news/5-largest-health-insurance-companies-by-membership.html

Value Line. 2020. "Investment Survey." Accessed March 13, 2020.

The Complex World of University Healthcare Systems

Centers for Medicare & Medicaid Service. 2019. "National Health Expenditure Data: Historical." Last modified December 17, 2019. https://www.cms.gov/Research-Statistics-Data-and-Systems/Statistics-Trends-and-Reports/NationalHealthExpendData/NationalHealthAccountsHistorical

Stanford Healthcare. n.d. "Consolidated Financial Statements and Accompanying Consolidating Information: August 31, 2019 and 2018." PDF file. Accessed June 8, 2020. https://stanfordhealthcare.org/about-us/bondholder-general-financial-information/audited-financial-statements.html

Stanford University. n.d. "Stanford University Annual Financial Report: August 31, 2019 and 2018." PDF file. Accessed June 8, 2020. https://bondholder-information.stanford.edu/pdf/SU_AnnualFinancialReport_2019.pdf

U.C. Office of the President. n.d. "University of California Revenue and Expense Trends: Fiscal Years 2010 through 2014." PDF file, University of California (website). Accessed June 8, 2020. https://finreports.universityofcalifornia.edu/index.php?file=retrends/retrends_2014.pdf

—. n.d. "University of California Revenue and Expense Trends: Fiscal Years 2015 through 2019." PDF file, University of California (website). Accessed June 8, 2020. https://finreports.universityofcalifornia.edu/index.php?file=retrends/retrends_2019.pdf

University of Colorado. n.d. "University of Colorado: 2019 Annual Financial Report." PDF file. Accessed June 8, 2019. https://www.cu.edu/doc/2019cuafrpdf

University of Texas System. n.d. "The University of Texas System Consolidated Financial Statements for the Years Ended August 31, 2019 and 2018 and Independent Auditors' Report." PDF file, University of Texas System

(website). Accessed June 8, 2020.
https://www.utsystem.edu/sites/default/files/do
cuments/report-state/2020/consolidated-
annual-financial-report-fy-2019/ut-system-
audit-afr-2019.pdf

Yale University. n.d. "Financial Report 2018–2019."
PDF file. Accessed June 8, 2020.
https://your.yale.edu/sites/default/files/annual-
report-2018-2019.pdf

The Piñata of Healthcare: The Pharmaceutical Industry

Centers for Disease Control and Prevention. n.d.
"Table 36: Emergency Department Visits
Within the Past 12 Months among adults aged
18 and over, by Selected Characteristics:
United States, Selected Years 1997–2017."
PDF file. Accessed June 8, 2020.
https://www.cdc.gov/nchs/data/hus/2018/036.p
df

—. n.d. "Table 39: Persons with Hospital Stays in the
Past Year, by Selected Characteristics: United
States, Selected Years 1997–2017." PDF file.
Accessed June 8, 2020.
https://www.cdc.gov/nchs/data/hus/2018/039.p
df

Centers for Medicare & Medicaid Service. 2019.
"National Health Expenditure Data:

Historical." Last modified December 17, 2019.
https://www.cms.gov/Research-Statistics-Data-and-Systems/Statistics-Trends-and-Reports/NationalHealthExpendData/NationalHealthAccountsHistorical

Department of Health and Human Services. 2016. "ASPE Issue Brief: Observations on Trends in Prescription Drug Spending." PDF file. Last modified March 8, 2016. https://aspe.hhs.gov/system/files/pdf/187586/Drugspending.pdf

Kirzinger, Ashley, Lunna Lopes, Bryan Wu, and Mollyann Brodie. 2019. "KFF Health Tracking Poll–February 2019: Prescription Drugs." Kaiser Family Foundation (website). Last modified March 1, 2019. https://www.kff.org/health-cf93osts/poll-finding/kff-health-tracking-poll-february-2019-prescription-drugs/

Shahbandeh, M. 2019 "Total Number of Retail Prescriptions Filled Annually in the U.S. 2013–2025." Last modified November 12, 2019. https://www.statista.com/statistics/261303/total-number-of-retail-prescriptions-filled-annually-in-the-us/

The Pharmaceutical Industry's Conundrum

Centers for Medicare & Medicaid Service. 2019. "National Health Expenditure Data: Historical." Last modified December 17, 2019. https://www.cms.gov/Research-Statistics-Data-and-Systems/Statistics-Trends-and-Reports/NationalHealthExpendData/NationalHealthAccountsHistorical

Congress.gov. 2003. "H.R.1 - Medicare Prescription Drug, Improvement, and Modernization Act of 2003." Last modified December 8, 2003. https://www.congress.gov/bill/108th-congress/house-bill/1

Cubanski, Juliette, Tricia Neuman, Sarah True, and Meredith Freed. 2019. "What's the Latest on Medicare Drug Price Negotiations?" Kaiser Family Foundation (website). Last modified October 17, 2019. https://www.kff.org/medicare/issue-brief/whats-the-latest-on-medicare-drug-price-negotiations/

McKesson. 2018. "Four Trends Shaping the Retail Pharmacy Business." Last modified August 20, 2018. https://www.mckesson.com/blog/retail-pharmacy-trends-to-watch/

United States Census Bureau. n.d. "2017 National Population Projections Tables: Main Series." Accessed June 8, 2020.

https://www.census.gov/data/tables/2017/demo
/popproj/2017-summary-tables.html

—. 2004. "Statistical Abstract of the United States:
2004–2005." Last modified August 26, 2004.
https://www.census.gov/library/publications/20
04/compendia/statab/124ed.html

USAFacts Institute. n.d. "10-K Report for the Fiscal
Year Ended September 30, 2017." PDF file.
Accessed June 8, 2020.
https://usafactscms.azureedge.net/media/docu
ments/USAFacts_Master_-
_Clean_FINAL_v2_41420_-_4-
16_9.37AM_update.pdf

Accessing Medicine Like the Rest of the World

Belson, Ken. 2018. "In Atlanta, Concessions Prices
Go Down and Revenue Goes Up." The New
York Times (website). Last modified January
25, 2018.
https://www.nytimes.com/2018/01/25/sports/fo
otball/nfl-concessions.html

OECD. 2020. "Pharmaceutical Spending: Indicator."
Accessed June 1, 2020.
https://data.oecd.org/healthres/pharmaceutical-
spending.htm

Ways and Means Committee Staff. 2019. "A Painful
Pill to Swallow: U.S. vs. International

Prescription Drug Prices." PDF file. Last modified September 2019. https://waysandmeans.house.gov/sites/democrats.waysandmeans.house.gov/files/documents/U.S.%20vs.%20International%20Prescription%20Drug%20Prices_0.pdf

Ode to the Bioscientists Fighting Cancer

Fink, Laurence D. 2013. "Longevity in the Age of Twitter: A Conversation with Laurence D. Fink, CEO of BlackRock." Video, 55:48. Filmed May 7, 2013. https://www.youtube.com/watch?time_continue=1&v=0Fdd9ULVVoA

Harding, Michael C., Chantel D. Sloan, Ray M. Merrill, Tiffany M. Harding, Brian J. Thacker, and Evan L. Thacker. 2018. "Transitions from Heart Disease to Cancer as the Leading Cause of Death in US States, 1999–2016." *Preventing Chronic Disease* 15 (December). doi: 10.5888/pcd15.180151.

Tang, J., A. Shalabi, and V.M. Hubbard-Lucey. 2018. "Comprehensive Analysis of the Clinical Immuno-Oncology Landscape." *Annals of Oncology* 29, no. 1 (January): 84–91. doi: 10.1093/annonc/mdx755.

Weir, Hannah K., Robert N. Anderson, Sallyann M. Coleman King, Ashwini Soman, Trevor D.

Thompson, Yuling Hong, Bjorn Moller, and
Steven Leadbetter. 2016. "Heart Disease and
Cancer Deaths—Trends and Projections in the
United States, 1969–2020." *Preventing
Chronic Disease* 13 (November). doi:
10.5888/pcd13.160211.

Xu, Jiaquan, Sherry L. Murphy, Kenneth D.
Kochanek, and Elizabeth Arias. n.d. "NCHS
Data Brief: Mortality in the United States,
2018." PDF file, Centers for Disease Control
and Prevention. Accessed June 8, 2020.
https://www.cdc.gov/nchs/products/databriefs/
db355.htm

The $2 Trillion Healthcare Bill

Leatherby, Lauren. 2016. "Medical Spending Among
the U.S. Elderly." JournalistsResource.org.
Last modified February 22, 2016.
https://journalistsresource.org/studies/governm
ent/health-care/elderly-medical-spending-
medicare/

United States Census Bureau. n.d. "2017 National
Population Projections Tables: Main Series."
Accessed June 8, 2020.
https://www.census.gov/data/tables/2017/demo
/popproj/2017-summary-tables.html

The Big Bucks Separating U.S. Healthcare from the Rest of the World

Centers for Medicare & Medicaid Service. 2019. "National Health Expenditure Data: Historical." Last modified December 17, 2019. https://www.cms.gov/Research-Statistics-Data-and-Systems/Statistics-Trends-and-Reports/NationalHealthExpendData/NationalHealthAccountsHistorical

OECD. n.d. "About." Accessed June 1, 2020. https://www.oecd.org/about/members-and-partners/

—. 2020. "Health Spending: Indicator." Accessed June 1, 2020. https://data.oecd.org/healthres/health-spending.htm

—. n.d. "Life Expectancy at Birth: Indicator." Accessed June 1, 2020. https://data.oecd.org/healthstat/life-expectancy-at-birth.htm

Xu, Jiaquan, Sherry L. Murphy, Kenneth D. Kochanek, and Elizabeth Arias. n.d. "NCHS Data Brief: Mortality in the United States, 2018." PDF file, Centers for Disease Control and Prevention. Accessed June 8, 2020. https://www.cdc.gov/nchs/products/databriefs/db355.htm

Healthcare Around the World

Frayer, Lauren. 2018. "U.K. Hospitals Are Overburdened, but the British Love Their Universal Health Care." NPR (website). Last modified March 7, 2018. https://www.npr.org/sections/parallels/2018/03/07/591128836/u-k-hospitals-are-overburdened-but-the-british-love-their-universal-health-care

Lieber, Dov. 2019. "Israel Prepares to Unleash AI on Health Care." The Wall Street Journal (website). Last modified September 15, 2019. https://www.wsj.com/articles/israel-prepares-to-unleash-ai-on-health-care-11568599261?mod=searchresults&page=1&pos=8

OECD. 2020. "Health Spending: Indicator." Accessed June 1, 2020. https://data.oecd.org/healthres/health-spending.htm

—. n.d. "Life Expectancy at Birth: Indicator." Accessed June 1, 2020. https://data.oecd.org/healthstat/life-expectancy-at-birth.htm

—.Stat. n.d. "Social Protection." Accessed June 1, 2020.

https://stats.oecd.org/Index.aspx?DataSetCode
=HEALTH_PROT

Otake, Tomoko. 2017. "Japan's Buckling Health Care
System at a Crossroads." The Japan Times
(website). Last modified February 19, 2017.
https://www.japantimes.co.jp/news/2017/02/19
/national/japans-buckling-health-care-system-
crossroads/#.Xtqwo2pKh0s

Tikkanen, Roosa, Robin Osborn, Elias Mossialos, Ana
Djordjevic, and George A. Wharton. 2020.
"International Healthcare System Profiles:
Israel." The Commonwealth Fund (website).
Last modified June 5, 2020.
https://international.commonwealthfund.org/co
untries/israel/

—. 2020. "International Healthcare System Profiles:
Japan." The Commonwealth Fund (website).
Last modified June 5,
2020.https://www.commonwealthfund.org/inte
rnational-health-policy-center/countries/japan

—. 2020. "International Healthcare System Profiles:
Switzerland." The Commonwealth Fund
(website). Last modified June 5, 2020.
https://www.commonwealthfund.org/internatio
nal-health-policy-center/countries/switzerland

University of Pennsylvania Leonard Davis Institute of
Health Economics. 2014. "An Overview of
Israel's Universal Health Care System." Last
modified August 2014.

https://ldi.upenn.edu/news/overview-israels-universal-health-care-system

Conclusion

Centers for Medicare & Medicaid Service. 2019. "National Health Expenditure Data: Historical." Last modified December 17, 2019. https://www.cms.gov/Research-Statistics-Data-and-Systems/Statistics-Trends-and-Reports/NationalHealthExpendData/NationalHealthAccountsHistorical

—. 2019. "National Health Expenditure Data: Projected." Last modified April 15, 2020. https://www.cms.gov/Research-Statistics-Data-and-Systems/Statistics-Trends-and-Reports/NationalHealthExpendData/NationalHealthAccountsProjected

Cohen, Robin A., Diane M. Makuc, Amy B. Bernstein, and Linda T. Bilheimer. 2009. "Health Insurance Coverage Trends, 1959–2007: Estimates from the National Health Survey." PDF file, *National Health Statistics Reports*, no. 17. Last modified July 1, 2009. https://www.cdc.gov/nchs/data/nhsr/nhsr017.pdf

Cohen, Robin A., Emily Terlizzi, and Michael E. Martinez. 2019. "Health Insurance Coverage:

Early Release of Estimates from the National Health Interview Survey, 2018." PDF file, Centers for Disease Control and Prevention (website). Last modified May 2019. https://www.cdc.gov/nchs/data/nhis/earlyreleas e/insur201905.pdf

United States Census Bureau. n.d. "Table 2: Projected Age and Sex Composition of the Population." Excel file, 2017 National Population Projections Tables. Accessed June 8, 2020. https://www.census.gov/data/tables/2017/demo /popproj/2017-summary-tables.html

Acknowledgments

To all the good folks who have deep care and the curiosity to create a better healthcare system.

About the Author

Stu Rodnick is a data fiend and pragmatist. His interest in healthcare economics developed as he became amazed by the advancements in the field of medicine (especially biotechnology) and dismayed by the many obstacles sitting between healthcare innovations and patients. He has broad interests and is a big fan of comedy and history.